This book is dedicated to every person who has battled with their own body and self-image. Everyone who is tired of not being on the outside who they know themselves to be on the inside. You are beautiful—let the world see you shine!

This book is also dedicated to the person who loved me 20 pounds ago and would love me no matter what I weigh: my husband, Stephen. I love you!

Table of Contents

Foreword

There is no shortage of dietary advice in the media today. However, every once in a while, a book comes along that just makes a lot of sense. *The UnDiet* is one of the funniest, most to-the-point books I have read in years. Instead of the usual questions of "What can't I eat? What do I have to give up?" this book approaches food for what it is: fun, tasty, and an integral part of life. No matter how you eat, you will find examples of small, realistic changes that can add up to real weight loss over the long term.

In this day of fast food, super-sized meals, food at every gathering, and limited physical activity, it may also be important to answer the obvious question: "Am I really hungry?" Somehow this book makes it seem simple to answer that question and then act accordingly.

Lynne M. Ausman, D.Sc., R.D.
Professor of Nutritional Biochemistry
Friedman School of Nutrition Science and Policy
Tufts University, Medford and Boston, MA

Chapter One

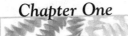

Learn from the Sumo Wrestlers

*How Eating More Frequently
Can Change Your Body
Composition for the Better*

Sure, we have all spent many a day pondering the secrets of weight loss. However, what about weight gain? Have you ever thought about the secrets to weight *gain*? Perhaps if we knew how to successfully gain weight and maintain that weight we could deduce the path to losing it. And guess what? You're in luck. I just happen to know the secret to gaining weight.

One Big Meal

Sumo wrestlers. You know, the ones from Japan. Their whole career revolves around being fat, maintaining their fat, and of course, getting fatter. So let's study their diet for a minute. It's a very, very simple one. In fact, would you believe they only eat once a day? That's right, one huge meal. Why? I'm telling you, they're smarter than they look.

You see Sumo wrestlers know that eating infrequently, like one or two big meals a day as opposed to smaller, more frequent meals, lowers our metabolism. Now once you have a low metabolism you're well on your way to being fat. That means your body burns calories at a rate that is slower than normal, which of course is good if you are a Sumo wrestler. This is why it's been found that most obese Americans do not eat breakfast, and eat two or fewer meals a day. Think about the people you know who struggle with weight—how often do they eat?

> Sumo wrestlers know that eating infrequently... lowers our metabolism.

Conversely, this is why most "naturally thin" (whatever that means) people eat three meals a day, and snack often. You see, every time we eat, we raise our metabolism, so the best way to have a fast metabolism is to eat small, frequent meals and snacks. But here's the big disclaimer: eat only when you're hungry and stop when you are full.

Most of us were raised to think snacking was "bad," and perhaps rightly so when our version of a snack was a bag of chips and a soda. But of course, a snack can also be a piece of fruit and a handful of sunflower seeds. The point is that snacking is neither good nor bad in and of itself. When we're hungry, a snack is good because it keeps our metabolism up and running. When we're hungry and we don't eat, it is bad because it lowers our metabolism. Moreover, when we're not hungry and we eat—well, we all know that's just plain overeating.

> When we're hungry and don't eat, it lowers our metabolism.

No Fattening Foods

Okay, now that all your former perceptions have been turned upside down, let me throw you a real whopper (no, not a Burger King Whopper—that's just where your mind is at). You ready? *There is no such thing as fattening food.* Now hear me out. I'm not saying there is no such thing as food that's high in fat, obviously there's plenty of that. However, what I am declaring is that high-fat food is not the same thing as "fattening" food. Why? Because no food in itself is fattening, but instead it's the way we *eat* the food. If we eat only when hungry and stop when we're full, nothing is fattening!

> No food in itself is fattening, but instead it's the way we eat the food.

Check it out. Let's say we find two half-starved people (for the point of discussion, they're equally half-starved), and we give each of them an unlimited amount of food. To the first, we'll give nonfat pretzel sticks; to the second, good old naturally high in fat cashews. Now we tell these people to eat until they are satisfied and then stop. Who do you think will eat the most food? Of course, the pretzel guy will eat more. The poor guy will probably go through three or four boxes of pretzels before he's even remotely full. The lucky cashew person will have stopped eating long ago. In fact, he probably ate a cup of cashews and he's on his way back home. The amazing thing is that they will both have eaten the same amount of calories! Therefore, neither will have gained weight!

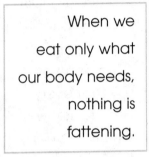

When we eat only what our body needs, nothing is fattening.

Get it? Everything is "fattening" when it's in excess, yet when we eat only what our body needs, nothing is fattening. That means eating at least three meals a day and often it requires having snacks.

How to be Naturally Thin

I once had a "naturally thin" roommate, who incidentally was also very beautiful, and I, as women often do, liked to study what Carolyn ate. I was also in good physical shape—but I exercised! She didn't even work for it! For the most part, Carolyn ate healthy food. But what I learned most of all was that it wasn't so much *what* she ate, as *how* she ate. The woman was an all-out snacker! She'd often sit down to a meal, find herself full in the middle of it, and then finish it off several hours later. So even her "meals" were more like snacks. One time the two of us drove together from California to Colorado, and I've never recalled stopping at so many gas stations—just for snacks! Sometimes candy, sometimes nuts, dried fruit, or sunflower seeds, but always snacks. Actually, I know some people who went on a trip to Europe with Carolyn after college, and they later confided that she was a wonderful travel companion but they sure got tired of stopping in small villages in search of snacks.

> I can honestly say that every person I know who is "naturally thin"…is a snacker.

In fact, I can honestly say that every person I know who is "naturally thin" (I still don't know quite what that means) is not an exercise-aholic, a weight lifter, or a diet expert, but a *snacker*. They have this innate ability to sense when they are hungry, eat, and then stop when they're full. It can slow down your travel plans, but I'd say it's well worth it.

Simple, right? Simple and small, but so important. And that's the key, small, simple changes—*not cold turkey ones.*

Chapter Two

Let's Talk
Cold Turkey

*Diets Don't Work but Baby
Steps Do, Especially When It Comes
to the Sneakiest Calories*

*E*veryone who has ever attempted to change bad habits knows that "baby steps" are essential. Little by little, those incremental changes add up, and the goal is finally reached. In contrast, going "cold turkey" is not only traumatic and painful, but often downright impossible. Common knowledge, right? Wrong. At least that is when we're talking about eating.

Although we've made progress in changing many harmful behaviors, when it comes to diet, Americans are still in cold turkey mode.

When most of us talk about losing weight, we talk about making a drastic change in the way we eat— called a diet. While it's possible to lose a tremendous amount of weight on a diet, the problem is it never stays off. That's because diets don't work, due to their very nature. The essence of a diet is to make a serious restriction in the calories we consume. It's strenuous and severe, like running a marathon for which we haven't trained. It's definitely a cold turkey experience—where we're counting down the days (or pounds) to our goal.

> Dieting is like running a marathon for which we haven't trained.

Yet here's the problem: once those pounds have been shed, what happens? We're faced with two distasteful options. Either we return to our regular eating pattern and gain back all that weight again, or we stay on the loathsome diet forever, but stay trim. Hmmm… decisions, decisions.

In fact, the only way a diet can work is if we stay on it forever. As soon as we deviate back to our normal behavior, our body returns to its former size. And why not? We don't expect to continually receive paychecks from a job we've left, so why expect to maintain weight loss from a diet we've quit!

Baby Steps

One of the best ways to lose weight is by cutting back a small amount of calories, every day. The key words here are *small* and *every day*. Why? Because it's realistic. When we reduce our calories by an amount that's hardly noticeable, we are able to stick with it for the long haul, and that's where it adds up.

> We can lose weight by cutting back a small amount of calories— every day.

For example, say we decide we can realistically commit to forgoing a measly 100 calories, every day. It could hardly be called a sacrifice, and in fact, most of us wouldn't know the difference (100 calories is about 3 percent of the typical American diet). But here's the math: one pound of body fat is made up of 3,500 calories, therefore, losing 100 calories from our diet each day will cause us to drop a pound every 35 days. Now this may seem slow, but remember, it's not a diet but a *lifestyle change*. Thus, over a period of two years, we can expect to lose 20 pounds—with hardly an effort. Better yet, it's permanent. Now time is no longer the enemy as with a cold turkey diet, where we're counting down days and minutes. Instead, time is working *for* us. It's on our side!

> Losing 100 calories from our diet each day will cause us to drop a pound every 35 days.

And we can go on. If we were to reduce our daily calorie intake by 200 calories (still a miniscule amount), we could expect to lose a pound every 17 days, and 40 pounds over two years. Again, it's permanent weight loss because it is small and therefore can be continued forever.

Your First Baby Step

Okay, now that I've got you convinced, how do you start? Again, it's simple. For starters, you can stop drinking beverages besides water. You've heard repeatedly how important it is to drink eight glasses of water a day. But did you ever learn why? Water is an essential nutrient for a healthy body, just like any other vitamin or mineral. Only water filters the kidneys, carries nutrients through the bloodstream, and hydrates our cells. When we are even slightly dehydrated, which many of us are without being aware of it, we can experience fatigue, headache, and (gasp) a false sense of hunger.

> When we are even slightly dehydrated...we can experience a false sense of hunger.

New studies are showing a myriad of benefits of drinking enough water, which incidentally, most of us do not do. Some of these benefits include preventing cancer, ridding the body of toxic wastes, fighting off headache and fatigue, and yes—even weight loss. One study even documented an obese woman who lost 42 pounds in 18 months simply by following a program that included a substantial increase in water consumption. One of the reasons it's believed drinking water causes weight loss is because we often confuse our body's need for hydration with food. Personally, I can testify that I've found myself thinking of food when what I really needed was water. I remember one time I was about to reach for the cupboard when it occurred to me: "I don't think I'm hungry, but thirsty!" After I downed that glass of cold water I realized I was right!

> We often confuse our body's need for hydration with food.

Another reason drinking enough water (at least 64 oz a day) has been linked to weight loss is because it's necessary for the proper functioning of the kidneys. One study at the University of Utah found that dehydration—something that most Americans are chronically experiencing—leads to a lowered metabolism. It was found that by drinking enough water we allow our kidneys to function at maximum capacity, which incidentally means our liver doesn't have to help the kidneys do their job. When the liver is freed from being an aid to the kidneys, it is able to focus on its own tasks, one of which is the proper metabolism of fat! So, in

> When our kidneys receive enough water, our liver is able to break down fat properly.

other words, if you want your body to efficiently break down fat rather than storing it, you need to do your part in drinking enough water!

The Sneakiest Calories

It's not only that water itself is so amazing, but *replacing* other beverages with water cuts out zillions of calories. In fact, the only place we should get calories from is food—never from drinks. The reason? The calories from beverages don't make us full, as do food calories. When we chew food, the mechanical motion of our jaw and tongue sends a message to the brain that says, "I'm eating and becoming satisfied." When we *drink* calories, there's no such communication, and therefore we continue to eat even after we've consumed the calories we need. Think about it, when was the last time you heard someone say, "I'm hungry. I'm going to go drink a soda"?

Need more proof? One study at Purdue University had volunteers eat 450 calories' worth of jellybeans every day for a month and keep a record of everything else they ate. At the month's end, the jellybeans were replaced with 450 calories of daily soda (a little less than three cans). Researchers found that while the volunteers had consumed the jellybeans, they had eaten smaller meals because they were naturally more full. During the jellybean period, they didn't gain weight.

> Soft drinks are the fifth largest source of calories for adults.

Yet when they switched to soda, volunteers gained weight (and how!) because their appetites, and diets, returned to normal, while they still took in an additional 450 calories a day. That's significant, especially considering that in the U.S., soft drinks are the *fifth* largest source of calories for adults! That's including all other foods, solid and liquid.

So by simply replacing one glass of juice, soda, milk, iced tea, café mocha, or whatever your beverage of choice may happen to be, with one glass of water, you're on your way to permanent weight loss—if you stick with it. Let's say you decide to cut out one can of soda a day (good choice! But be forewarned: soda is addictive!), that's 150 calories lost every day. That's between 10 and 15 pounds shed a year—from just that tiny change. And of course, by kicking the soda habit altogether, you are going to see greater results, faster, but just be sure you're committed for the long haul.

> By cutting out one can of soda a day... that's between 10-15 pounds shed a year.

More Amazing Stories

Once, as I was teaching on this subject in a college nutrition class, I had a young male student interrupt me, waving his hand fervently. He said, "Ms. Schweigerdt, you are totally right about this. I'd like to share what happened to me. A couple years ago, I was drinking four or five cans of soda a day and, needless to say, I was overweight. Then I decided to stop drinking soda altogether and switch to water. The first month I did this, I lost 25 pounds. The second month, I lost another 20 pounds. I stuck with it for a year or so, but then began to drink only lemonade. I gained back all that weight in no time. Again, I switched back to water and in a few months dropped those 45 pounds."

> Let's quit the cold turkey diets and start with some baby steps!

Are you inspired? Let's quit the cold turkey diets and start with some baby steps! Just for further inspiration, think about the Grand Canyon for a second. If you've ever been to this national monument, you were probably amazed to realize that steep canyon walls over two vertical miles down were made not by an earthquake nor an iceberg, but simply by a steady stream of water—*over time*. Each and every day as the Colorado River flowed, it carved out a path just a tiny bit deeper into the ground. That's what it's all about, small changes over a long time. If that doesn't do it for you, think of how a pregnant woman needs to gain weight.

She is advised to gain an average of 30 pounds before her due date. Many newly pregnant women think this gives them the liberty to pig out for the duration of their pregnancy. Unfortunately, it doesn't. In fact, to gain those 30 pounds,

> That's what it's all about, small changes over a long time.

they are recommended to increase their food intake by a mere 300 calories a day! How disheartening! That's the equivalent of an extra whole-wheat bagel (minus the topping) or a half-cup serving of raisins a day! (Incidentally, it's also the equivalent of two cans of soda). Yet again, *over time*—nine months to be exact— that little bit of extra food will add up to produce, well, a baby.

What About Diet Soda?

But maybe the question is crossing your mind, "What about diet soda? That has only one calorie. How can cutting that out help me lose weight?" You're in luck. I happen to know another secret: artificial sweeteners (including those in diet drinks) have actually been documented by the American Cancer Society as causing people to gain more weight than those who do not use them.

How's that? When your mouth tastes the sweet flavor of artificial sweeteners, it sends the brain a message: "Sugar is coming down the pipes!" Therefore, the pancreas is alerted to secrete into the blood the notorious hormone called insulin. The insulin then waits in the blood… and waits, but no sugar comes. So then, the brain gets another message—the message that there's no sugar but lots of insulin, and that creates an urgent craving for sugar and simple

> Artificial sweeteners create an urgent craving for sugar and simple carbohydrates.

28

(refined, or processed) carbohydrates. In other words, it makes you want to eat junk food, right now!

Think about this—how many people do you know who have actually lost weight using artificial sweeteners? I've never heard of any. In fact, the people I see using artificial sweeteners are usually quite overweight. Obviously, the sweeteners aren't quite living up to their promises, now are they?

What If I Don't Like Water?

Another dilemma you might have with the replacing-beverages-with-water idea is that you don't like drinking water! If that's how you feel, you're not alone. Not only are soda and other beverages addictive because they contain artificial flavors and colors that act as chemicals in the brain, but over time, they make it very difficult for you to enjoy a real, natural beverage, like water.

Well, let me assure you that in the beginning, I didn't like drinking water either. It takes time to re-establish a taste for what is wholesome and natural, especially when we've been drinking junk beverages since our earliest years. But here's how to begin. Get a water pitcher that filters water and store it in your fridge. If the only water option is tap water that tastes bad and is room temperature, your efforts to drink only water will not last long, I assure you. Add slices of lemon, orange, or lime to your water for flavor. Boil water and make tea (regular or herbal—my favorite is peppermint). Hot water, like tea, is especially helpful because it fills you up and takes longer for your body to digest. This is also true for foods like soups.

> It takes time to re-establish a taste for what is wholesome and natural.

Besides, tea—regular and herbal—is good for you. It took some time, but after a few months of slowly weaning myself off juice and other drinks and replacing them with water, I actually got to the place where all I want to drink is water! It's truly more thirst quenching than anything else!

Chapter Three

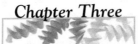

It's Not Just What You Eat...

"You Are What You Eat" Is Only Half the Story: How Fibrous Food Causes Weight Loss—Literally

You have counted calories, you have counted fat, and, more recently, you have counted carbohydrates, but none of them cause weight loss. Only food containing fiber causes weight loss—literally.

You see, when we think of weight loss and diets and such, the attention usually focuses on what we take in—as in calories. Rarely does it touch on the topic of what goes out, and when it does, we're usually talking about exercise. Exercise is essential to being healthy and losing weight or maintaining a healthy weight, don't get me wrong. In fact, I'm an exercise junkie. But what I'm getting at is that there's another way to increase the calories that go out (besides raising your metabolism), and that's to literally increase what goes out the other end of your digestive system. No, I'm not suggesting buying laxatives and purging your system. I'm talking about fiber.

> Foods high in fiber cause our body to burn more calories—and gain very few.

Foods that are high in fiber cause us to gain very few calories because, if you haven't noticed, much of it goes right out the back door.

For example, would you believe that for every gram of fiber we consume our body burns 7 calories during its digestion? That means that if we ate only the *minimum* recommended amount of fiber each day (25 g), we would burn off about 200 calories a day, which would add up to one pound every two weeks! That's potentially 24 pounds a year... and not from *decreasing* our food intake—just by switching it to more strategic foods!

Here's the paraphrased version of a quote I once read that summarizes this principle elegantly: "We are what we eat and we don't excrete." See, that old proverb that says we are what we eat is only half right! We will never be successful in attaining a healthy weight unless we take in the whole equation: calories in—calories out = calories stored (fat). So now let's look at those outgoing calories.

> We can lose weight not from decreasing our food intake—but by eating more fibrous foods.

Food—Minus the Calories

What if someone told you they discovered this new type of food that tastes great, expands in the stomach so it fills you up quickly, digests slowly so it keeps blood sugar from dropping and so you're not hungry for hours—and then after all this, that many of the food's calories aren't even absorbed but are excreted right out into the toilet? What would you say? "Where can I get this food?! What store carries it?" Well my friend, this food is actually not new at all, but has been around for thousands of years. It's called "high-fiber food," and it is only found in whole-plant foods.

These foods: fruits and vegetables, nuts and seeds, whole grains such as brown rice, oatmeal, popcorn, whole grain breads and cereals, and legumes, which include all varieties of beans, lentils and peas, are all significant sources of fiber. In the Old Testament in the Bible, breads were always made of whole grains, usually consisting of many different grains, such as flax, millet, barley, and rye. This is to say these foods have been around for quite some time. Yet, unfortunately, our modern Western diets have caused many of these foods to be altogether forgotten. Today's food industries take what was created as whole and perfect, and they process the heck out of

> High-fiber foods include popcorn, oatmeal, nuts and seeds...

it, causing the fiber as well as most of the foods' other nutrients to be lost.

The Carbohydrate Question

This brings us to the Carbohydrate Question. These days, everyone seems to be counting carbohydrates, with the belief that carbohydrates are what's making us fat in the first place. Many people I talk to about whole-plant foods and fiber ask, "But aren't those carbohydrates? Shouldn't I be limiting them?" Well this is another one of those half-truths.

> It's important to know the difference between "good" and "bad" carbohydrates.

Really, when you get down to it, there are two very distinct types of "carbohydrate" foods. (I say "carbohydrate" because in its natural state no food is pure carbohydrate, but a combination of protein, carbohydrate, and fat.)

The first type of carbohydrate is the kind we need to avoid with zeal. These are the processed or refined foods. They are essentially what man has made out of what was once a perfect, God-made food. These are your pre-prepared foods: in short, everything that comes in a box, a can, or a plastic bag. In other words: crackers, store-bought baked goods, chips, frozen dinners, fast foods, boxed macaroni and cheese, instant soups, puddings, cake and muffin mixes, canned soups and foods…you get the picture. They are also your "white" foods—white rice, breads, pasta noodles, and cereals made primarily from white flour. These foods were once whole-plant foods, but have been corrupted into low-fiber, low-nutrient, high-artificial-additive food. These foods are good for gaining weight, but never for losing it.

> Low-fiber, processed foods are good for gaining weight, but never for losing it.

On the other hand, all whole-plant foods are rich in fiber (remember this is key for outgoing calories) and many, many other nutrients. One of these nutrients is a trace mineral called chromium. You may have heard of chromium in relation to weight loss. Supplement companies often market chromium as a weight-loss agent. Again, this is a half-truth (the marketing industry is good at these). In reality, chromium does facilitate weight loss by reducing the appetite, but only if a person's diet is deficient in chromium. When we get enough chromium from our food, our appetite is healthy and normal. But when we eat too few foods containing chromium,

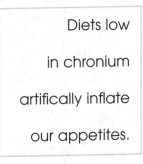

Diets low in chronium artifically inflate our appetites.

we develop an artificially elevated appetite. Since chromium only comes from whole-plant foods (not processed foods, and not meats, eggs, or dairy), no wonder it is estimated that a full 90 percent of Americans have diets deficient in chromium!

Much more needs to be said regarding the "low-carbohydrate diets." These diets are actually quite dangerous and result in rapid loss of calcium from the bones, as well as a high risk of kidney disease. I encourage you to do your own research on these diets if you know anyone who is on one.

The Only Win/Win Diet

So eating a diet rich in whole-plant foods is a win-win situation: you get your fiber and your chromium to boot. Calories in *and* calories out. Unfortunately, the average American woman gets less than half the recommended amount of fiber in her diet each day— only 12 grams. (It is recommended to have between 25 and 40 grams from food daily.) And when you think about it, no wonder we have such a weight problem! When we consume diets rich in processed foods, meats, eggs, and dairy, we are taking in plenty of calories, and we're keeping each and every one of them.

And I'm not the only one who's discovered this fantastic secret. Recently, a study at Harvard followed a group of 2900 people and their diets for ten years. They found that those with the diets lowest in fiber gained the most weight, and not surprisingly, were the most likely to develop risk factors for coronary heart disease. Conversely, the people with the highest fiber

> The people with the diets lowest in fiber gained the most weight.

diets gained the least weight and had the fewest risk factors. Particularly surprising about this study was that they found that fat intake made no difference in weight gain. In fact, those who gained the most weight were also the ones with the lowest fat diets!

> Those who gained the most weight were also the ones with the lowest fat diets.

So, if you thought nuts were fattening, think again. They're also high in fiber, which means many of the calories they give you are only passing through! What's more, many low-fat, nonfat, and reduced-fat foods actually have more calories than their natural counterparts do! It's a marketing ploy for food manufacturers to take out the fat, add more of the actual foods (like sugar, for flavor), and sell it as "low-fat." Sneaky, but hey, it works. Just another reason to avoid processed foods!

A Personal Note

Personally, I just have to share with you that changing my diet to include only whole-plant foods has caused me to lose weight—and I honestly wasn't even trying! (Not that I'm complaining now!) I had been a vegetarian for years and was happy with my weight and body size. It wasn't until I took out dairy products and replaced them with plant-based substitutes that I actually lost 20 pounds, slowly, over the course of a year. I decided to substitute milk with almond milk (a delicious alternative to soy or rice milk), and regular cheese to almond cheese. The milk I had been drinking before the switch was 1% fat. Almond milk is also 1% fat, although it does have fewer calories. But what I believe made the true difference is that the almond products have *fiber*. Granted, it's only 1 gram of fiber (milk, like all food from animal origins, has no fiber), but then again, that means I have a little more outgoing calories every day, and my body is burning 7 extra calories for that 1 gram of fiber! Remember, over time that adds up. It certainly did for me. It was a slow weight loss, and I didn't even feel deprived!

> Milk, like all food from animal origins, has no fiber.

Incidentally, my friend Kymm Griffin, who helped me edit this book, has also switched to a plant-based diet. (Reading this chapter over and over probably made its mark.) Since she has "made the switch," she's lost 24 pounds, and says she not only feels better than ever, but even has a much harder time working up a sweat when exercising! Just imagine! Kymm also found that she recovered significantly faster from a C-section when she was practicing her new eating habits, in contrast to her first C-section a few years prior. She said after the second she didn't need any pain medication, and was up and about shopping only a few days after her surgery!

> If you look at one thing on the food label, look at the fiber content.

Focus on the Fiber

So while the media, doctors, and dieticians are still talking about watching your fat, calories, or even carbohydrates, take it from me—just focus on the fiber. (That's catchy, isn't it?) If you look at one thing on the food label, look at the fiber content. The more, the better. But even a little is good. You don't even need to count it, just make sure that *everything* you eat has fiber. However, shoot for a cereal with 4 or 5 grams of fiber and buy bread that has no less than 3 fiber grams per slice. The fiber in your food will cause calories to be lost as they bind with the fiber. Taking a fiber supplement, such as Fibercon, will not do this because it does not bind with the actual food. Because no actual food is lost, all the calories will remain.

> The fiber in your food will cause calories to be lost as they bind with the fiber.

If you really want to be sure you're getting enough fiber, you'll be feeling it in the outgoing department of your digestive tract, if you catch my drift. In fact, you will soon notice that it takes you no longer to eliminate solid waste (scientifically referred to as "#2") than liquid, or "#1." Not only will this result in more bathroom efficiency, but it will also prevent or heal a multitude of colon diseases such as colon cancer, hemorrhoids, diverticulitis, constipation, and even irritable bowel syndrome!

Chapter Four

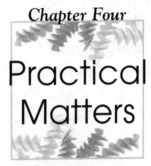

Practical Matters

***The Best "Fast Food," How to
Eat Defensively, and the Surprising
Truth about Restaurant Food***

So let's put some of this information together into a nifty application. Eating at least three small meals a day plus possibly snacks can be quite time-consuming. Or, if you choose to get your food from restaurants and vendors, it can be quite expensive (and usually not too high in fiber). Processed foods are too darn convenient and we've become dependent upon them.

So what to do? Here's what I do: I make my own "convenience" foods because I cook everything in bulk. I can't remember the last time I made a meal that lasted only for one evening. Everything I make is in grandscale—that way, when I'm hungry and don't feel like cooking, I don't have to. I just heat up one of the week's leftovers. These are meals like whole wheat pasta dishes, pizza, beans and brown rice, soups, stir-fry dishes, salads, etc. Also, I make sure to always have plenty of high fiber snacks on hand. This is easy, because most of them will store for long periods, such as nuts, sunflower and pumpkin seeds, trail mix, and dried fruit. Other fast-fiber snacks I make include fruit smoothies, hot oatmeal with raisins, stone ground tortilla chips with salsa, and fresh fruit in season.

> When I'm hungry and don't feel like cooking, I don't have to.

Meal or SUPERMeal?

Now, something needs to be said regarding what constitutes "a meal." Newsflash: did you know that today's restaurant servings are no longer considered "meals," but instead, "supermeals"?! That's right, since the 1970s alone, the average plate size used in restaurants has increased by a radius of two inches all around! Today's hamburgers, fries, tacos, chicken sandwiches, etc. are often double that of what they were less than 30 years ago!

Studies show that a typical meal at an ordinary American restaurant has 1,000 calories—and that's not including appetizer, drinks, or dessert! (Just for contrast, the average meal in a restaurant in France is between one-third to one-half the size of ours.) Considering that the average American eats out one-third of the time, that's a problem, especially when most of us were raised to "finish everything on our plates." And incidentally, according to The American Institute for Cancer Research, a whopping 67% of Americans eat everything on their plates—no matter how much is on it!

> A typical meal at an ordinary American restaurant has 1,000 calories.

So why is the restaurant industry so eager to give us all this extra food? Again, marketing. People see bigger sizes as better value—more for their money. It makes them more likely to choose one eating establishment over another. Unfortunately, it also is making them (us) fat.

I'll never forget the time I was sitting in a restaurant in O'Hare Airport. A woman seated at a table next to me was making her order, "I'll have the nacho plate please." The waitress then asked her what she would like for an appetizer—as if it was a "given" that she even wanted one! "I suppose I'll have the stuffed potato skins." When the appetizer plate was brought out, it was huge, to say the least. The woman, likely a graduate of the "finish everything on your plate" school, was only half way through the potato skins when the main dish arrived. She seemed surprised, remarking to the waitress, "This is a lot of food." She then proceeded to do her best at finishing the nachos. But what surprised me was that this woman didn't *expect*

> This woman didn't expect to be given enough food to feed a small army.

to be given enough food to feed a small army. After all, I'm sure it wasn't the first time it had happened.

But for some reason, most of us have never even considered that restaurant servings are no longer normal, but "superservings." Yet in order for us to attain a healthy weight, we must turn back the clock to the seventies and establish a new (old) standard of "normal."

> Excess food is wasted whether it's thrown out or added to our waistlines.

Today, appetizer plates are what we once considered as full meals. Main dishes are twice that big. Plus, most of us have a hard time leaving food on our plates. We worry that we're "wasting it." But I'll tell you the truth; *excess* food (no matter how "healthy" it is) is wasted whether it's being thrown out or added to our waistlines. Our becoming fatter is in no way going to help the hungry people of the world. Regarding junk food—how can there even be a question of wasting it? It's not food anyway: it's junk, and we all know the rightful place of junk is in the garbage.

How to Eat Out the Right Way

Yet there are even better solutions than throwing excess food away. One thing I've found to be helpful is to eat out less often! Would you believe it actually makes it more fun when you do? Suddenly, eating out becomes a treat; I'm saving tons of money—and calories. When I do go out, I go with the expectation that I will most likely only eat half my meal (because it will be twice the size of a "normal" meal). Often, I'll bring a recycled take-home box to the restaurant with me just for a reminder. Sometimes, I'll order only an appetizer or soup. The waiter will usually ask if I'd like something else with that, and I patiently reply, "First I'll see if I'm still hungry after I finish my appetizer, and if I am, I'll let you know."

> I go out with the expectation that I will most likely only eat half my meal.

Here's another new habit we need to begin: getting used to saying no. Actually, make that, "No thank you." Everywhere we go food constantly bombards us—low-fiber, processed, super-sized food, no less. In fact, it even comes right into our homes, doesn't it? What kind of commercials do we see on TV? Seven out of ten times, it's food (usually fast food). When we go to a party, meeting, or just about any social situation, what is almost always present? Food, soda, and more food. When you travel on an airplane, flight attendants parade up and down the aisle, offering snacks, soda, and low-fiber, processed meals. When we're invited to someone's house, what's the first thing they offer? "Would you like anything to eat or drink?" When we drive down the freeway, what signs jump out

> When we say *no* we must understand that we are not *missing out* in any way.

at us? Would you believe signs for restaurants that serve *food*? We live in a food-functioning society. And there's no way to change that. But we can change our response to it, by learning to "just say no."

No More "Missing Out"

Here's the trick: when we say no, we must understand that we are not "missing out" in any way. Nor are we denying ourselves something we want. In fact, it's just the opposite. We are actually just being choosy. We're saying no, not because we *can't* eat or drink what's being offered, but because we don't *want* to. And it's true, we don't. We don't *want* to be overweight, and we don't *want* to put junk into our precious bodies. Once we recognize that it's not a matter of can't—sure, we can eat whatever we want—but a *want-* issue, then we will be free to do what we truly want to do. You know as well as I that if we think we can't do something, we begin to think we want that very thing with all our hearts! And that's just what is happening with food.

> It's not because we *can't* eat what's being offered us— but we honestly don't *want* it.

Here's another new habit: stop making impulse decisions! Don't you know that's where all those Quickie Mart-type stores are getting their profits? Even normal supermarkets put their candy and gum up at the front of the checkout stands. They're expecting you to make impulse decisions—which aren't really decisions at all. In fact, almost every time you say yes to the countless offers of food given to you, you are making an impulse decision. You are choosing the food or drink out of habit, instead of hunger. We need to think critically, "Hmmm, is this really what I want to eat? Is it that good or should I hold out for something better? Am I even hungry?"

How to Eat Defensively

One way I make sure to avoid impulse decisions when I'm on the road is by always taking food with me. I take travel-friendly, high-fiber snacks (again: trail mix, nuts, seeds, dried fruit, and even tea bags), so when I find myself facing offers of food or drinks I don't want, I have my trusty alternatives, helping me say, "No, thank you". Also, I'll make sure I ask the self-reflective questions like, "Am I even hungry or am I just bored, anxious, restless, or lonely?"

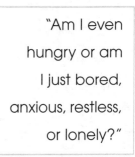

"Am I even hungry or am I just bored, anxious, restless, or lonely?"

Because this is at the root of our food-functioning society. Eating is not comfort. We may think it provides comfort, and surely, the industries that market their food products want us to believe this, but it never lives up to its promise. In fact, after we eat food to be comforted, we feel worse than before!

Love Your Food

One last new habit we need to learn: how to *savor* our food. Can I just share an interesting little tidbit? Most cultures in the world are very well practiced in savoring food. Food is a huge part of these cultures, as it is ours. But their attitude toward it is different. They simply love food. Most of these societies will dedicate hours each day to purchase, grow, or gather their food. Then they will spend many more hours preparing it. When they eat it, they almost always do so in the presence of many others: in an atmosphere of joy and celebration—daily! When they bite into their meal, they actually take the time to *taste* it. They are thankful as they savor the fragrance,

> Most cultures in the world take the time to actually taste their food.

aroma, and the flavor of each bite. In fact, the word for "tasty" or "delicious" in Spanish is *sabroso*, which means literally "to savor."

Nutrients are actually what give our food flavor, color, and aroma. The more nutrients, the more pleasing it is. Our bodies were designed to slowly savor the food we eat. The longer food

> Our bodies were designed to slowly savor the food we eat.

is on the tongue, the more saliva we secrete. Saliva is alkaline, and coats food before it's sent down into the extremely acidic stomach environment. The longer food remains in our mouth before it's swallowed, the less likely we are to develop ulcers! Also, as we chew our food, the brain receives the message that we are becoming satisfied. The longer we chew, the more satisfied we feel, and vice-versa.

What a contrast to the way we eat in our country today! Instead of slowly tasting and savoring each bite in the presence of friends and family, we are often in a hurry, eating over the sink or in a car—by ourselves. We hardly chew but instead think, "I've only got ten minutes so 'down the hatch.'" No wonder so many Americans have ulcers! I often wonder why people don't choose to eat healthier foods when they hardly taste what they're eating anyway! Yes, we are a culture that claims to love food, but our love-relationship has become quite dysfunctional.

> When you deliberately taste and enjoy each bite, you eat less.

Remember how I mentioned that in France portion sizes are often less than one-half that of ours? Yet, the French are world-renowned for *loving* food. They truly do, because they savor it. When you deliberately taste and enjoy each bite of your meal, you naturally eat less. You also eat more slowly, which allows your brain time to register that you are full. Ironically, even though the French diet is high in fat (although it's also much higher than ours in fiber) obesity rates are only one-fourth of what they are in the U.S. How unfair! They eat delicious food, spend oodles of time doing it, enjoy it more, and yet have much fewer weight problems than we do!

Trust My Mom

My mom has learned the art of savoring food—especially desserts. She actually recognizes the fantastic truth that *desserts aren't worth eating if you don't take time to taste them.* How profound! So what does she do? She almost always orders a dessert, but almost never finishes eating it! Why? "Because the first few bites are what taste the best anyway, and it's not like I'm still hungry at the end of my meal. I'm just eating it because I want something sweet at the end of my dinner. I'm a grown woman, and I don't have to clean my plate anymore!" What a delightful attitude. She has definitely conquered the "More is Better" lie. I'd almost say it's un-American!

> Desserts aren't worth eating if you don't take time to taste them.

So learn from my mom—or the French, Spanish, Asians, Africans, Indians, or Latin Americans—and slow down to taste and enjoy what you eat. When you go out to eat, make it a treat. Go to a restaurant where there is atmosphere: low lighting, comfy seats, quiet background, and of course, scrumptious food. When you eat at home, try to eat together with others, and do your best to make a calm, enjoyable environment. Eat only the food worth tasting; be choosy. Relax and savor each morsel. Give thanks for each bite, for not everyone in the world has as much food as we do. Eat with a thankful heart, and delight in the gift God has given you.

Chapter Five

How to Incorporate Painless Baby Steps into Your Life

A Bunch of Simple, Easy Ways to Lose Weight Without Denying Yourself or Good Food

Honestly, there are so many different types of baby steps to make in losing weight that my list in no way is exhaustive. Please feel free to invent your own: whatever fits your lifestyle and is easy for you. Also, you might be inspired by some of these suggestions to do something similar, but slightly different—do it!

Tea and Coffee Changes

One of the many ways I've caught myself drinking sneaky calories was through my daily tea-totaling. Knowing how good tea is for my body was one thing, but constantly adding honey for flavor wasn't part of the healthy plan. Unwittingly, I was adding countless calories to my diet every day just by adding honey (or sometimes sugar) to my twice-daily tea consumption! When I found a tea blend that I thought tasted great without sweetener (I recommend Good Earth tea), I was shaving off over 100 calories a day… which culminated in losing about four pounds in a month!

> Find a tea or coffee that is tasty without adding honey or sugar.

So if tea is part of your daily beverage, whether iced or hot, find one that is tasty without adding honey or sugar (and especially artificial sweetener!). The same goes for coffee. In my opinion, teas and coffees that are organically grown have much more flavor, and therefore don't need anything added. Remember that coffee and teas are diuretics, which mean they make your body lose more water than it should, and therefore contribute to dehydration (which impedes fat metabolism!), so drink these beverages in moderation and increase your water consumption to compensate.

> Coffee and tea contain no calories on their own except the calories we add with sugar & milk.

Also, if you don't feel you can go cold turkey by cutting out all sweeteners in your drinks, then try adding *less*! If you measure how much you add currently, and try to add only half of that, you'd make a significant difference in your calorie intake. You'll also find that your taste buds will acclimate to the less-sweet taste, so that eventually you may be able to completely cut out all sugar or honey.

In the same vein, you should know that coffee and tea contain no calories on their own, but it's only the calories we add through sugar, milk, cream, etc., that cause us to gain weight. No matter how small these additions may seem, they add up! So let's focus on the *other* calories: the dairy.

If you add milk or cream to coffee, and drink coffee regularly, you should know the *breakdown*:

For every two tablespoons of added…

- Cream—you gain 120 calories!
- Half & half—40 calories
- Whole milk—20 calories
- Reduced fat milk (2%)—17.5 calories
- Fat free milk—12.5 calories

Also, in exchange for these calories, you receive 0 grams of fiber.

Yet for two tablespoons of soy milk, you receive only 11 calories and a trace of fiber! And when we remember that each gram of fiber causes our body to burn 7 calories, we know that even *some* fiber is better than nothing, especially as it adds up.

Cereal Side-Note

Aside from dairy we add to coffee, the same applies to milk in our cereal. If you are thinking to yourself, "I only drink milk in my cereal," then think again. Those calories from milk, just like coffee, add up quickly, because they're part of your diet *every day*. So replacing milk with soy, rice, or almond milk will not only knock out calories but include fiber, which as we know, knocks out more calories!

> Replacing milk in cereal with soy, rice or almond milk will knock out calories.

For example, if you were to substitute 8 oz of reduced fat (2%) milk in your cereal every day with soy milk, you would result in a loss of 84 calories a day. If you switched from nonfat milk in your cereal to soy milk, you'd lose 40 calories a day. And that's not including the extra calories lost from the fiber! Also, this applies to yogurt, cheese, and ice cream. I will show the difference in calories and fiber for these—and many other foods—later in this section.

In fact, this switch alone is one of the major factors that helped me lose 20 pounds!

Coffee Drink Exposé

Okay, if you are one of the many Americans that have found yourself attracted to coffee drinks (you know, the café mochas, lattes, café au lait and cappacinos), there's a lot you need to know.

All of these drinks contain a high percentage of milk for their size, and unless you request otherwise, the milk is usually 2% fat.

For example, a normal-sized mocha (16 oz) is 12 oz, or three-fourths, pure milk! A normal 16 oz latte is also 12 oz milk, while a café au lait is 8 oz milk. A single cappacino, being only 6 oz, is 3 oz milk.

> A normal cafe mocha or latte contains 215 calories—all from milk!

Therefore, a normal mocha or latte contains approximately 215 calories—all from milk! If you were to have that milk replaced with nonfat soy milk, it'd only cost you 135 calories, not to mention 1 gram of fiber. So that's over 80 calories less—which again, adds up fast.

Another realistic baby step is to simply downsize (no, not down*load*) your normal servings of food. Now that you know that today's restaurants and fast food facilities serve not meals but Supermeals, you know to question your hunger and fullness when you go out, but this should be applied at home as well. If you were to truly stop eating when you are no longer hungry, the portions of your meals would probably drop off 100 calories easily. In addition, you might

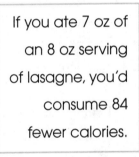

If you ate 7 oz of an 8 oz serving of lasagne, you'd consume 84 fewer calories.

have more of an appetite in between meals to snack, which would raise your metabolism!

For example, if you sat down to an 8 oz serving of homemade lasagna, and didn't finish it, but ate 7 oz, you would be kicking off 84 calories from your diet!

And of course, if that lasagna had been a high-fiber version (whole wheat noodles, vegetables, etc.), then you would be losing even more calories while becoming fuller, faster. So let's take a look at some of the countless high-fiber foods we have at our disposal:

Fruit

Medium apple with peel: 4 g fiber
Medium orange (no peel!): 4 g
Peach with peel: 3 g
Three small apricots: 6 g
Pear with peel: 4-5 g
Avocado (no peel!): 6 g
1 cup of dates: 13 g
1 cup of raisins: 5 g
10 dried figs: 17 g

Nuts/Seeds

1 cup almonds: 14 g
1 cup cashews: 4 g
1 cup macadamia nuts: 12 g

1 cup peanuts: 10 g

1 cup pistachios: 14 g

1 cup pumpkin seeds: 15 g

1 cup sunflower seeds: 8 g

1 cup walnuts: 6 g

2 tablespoons natural peanut butter: 3 g

Legumes and Vegetables

2/3 cup artichoke hearts: 6 g

1/2 cup black beans (cooked): 7 g

1/2 cup lima beans: 6 g

1/2 cup pinto beans: 7 g

1 cup cooked broccoli: 5 g

1 medium raw carrot: 2 g

1 ear of corn: 2 g

1 cup garbanzo beans (chickpeas): 8 g

1 cup kidney beans: 16 g

1/2 cup lentils: 5 g

1 cup navy beans: 16 g

1/2 cup black-eyed peas: 6 g

1 cup snow peas: 4 g

1 sweet yellow bell pepper: 4 g

1 medium potato with skin: 5 g (w/o skin: 2 g)
1 cup sundried tomatoes: 7 g

Whole Grains

1 cup barley (cooked): 8 g
1 cup oatmeal: 4 g
1 cup bulgar: 8 g
1 cup buckwheat flour: 7 g
1 cup brown rice: 4 g
1 cup whole wheat spaghetti noodles: 6 g
5 cups popcorn: 6 g
1 slice whole grain bread: 3-4 g
1 whole wheat bagel: 2-3 g
1 cup whole grain cereal: 4-5 g
1 oz stone ground corn tortilla chips: 3-4 g
1 whole wheat tortilla: 2-3 g
1 small corn tortilla: 2 g

Another easy "baby step" is to simply substitute foods that are low in fiber (and usually high in calories) with high fiber plant foods. Here are some examples of the difference in calories and fiber (and remember, fiber means 7 fewer total calories per gram!):

- 8 oz of homemade lasagna with meat: 382 calories, 3 g fiber
- 8 oz of homemade lasagna with no meat (extra vegetables): 298 calories, 5 g fiber
- *Difference*: 84 calories, 2 g fiber

- 1 oz Monterey Jack cheese: 100 calories, no fiber
- 1 oz Monterey Jack flavored almond cheese: 55 calories, 2 g fiber
- *Difference*: 45 calories, 2 g fiber

- 2 oz Jimmy Dean sausage: 250 calories, no fiber
- 2 oz Jimmy Dean 50% Less Fat sausage: 170 calories, no fiber
- 2 oz Gimme Lean Soy Sausage: 50 calories, 2 g fiber
- *Difference*: either 200 or 120 calories and 2 g fiber

- 1 serving 99% fat-free turkey slices: 60 calories, no fiber
- 1 serving Smart Deli Soy turkey slices: 40 calories, no fiber
- *Difference*: 20 calories

- 1 cup regular vanilla ice cream: 357 calories, no fiber
- 1 cup Soy Delicious vanilla ice cream: 260 calories, 2 g fiber
- *Difference*: 93 calories, 2 g fiber

- 4 oz lean burger patty: 316 calories, no fiber
- 1 Boca Burger (soy) patty: 130 calories, 5 g fiber
- *Difference*: 186 calories, 5 g fiber

- 8 oz peach yogurt: 190 calories, no fiber
- 8 oz peach soy yogurt: 190 calories, 1 g fiber
- *Difference*: 1 g fiber

- 3 oz potato chips: 480 calories, 3 g fiber
- 3 oz stone ground red corn tortilla chips: 420 calories, 12 g fiber
- *Difference*: 60 calories, 9 g fiber

- 3.5 oz bag of Cheetos: 560 calories, no fiber
- 5 cups homemade popcorn (no butter): 100 calories, 6 g fiber
- *Difference*: 460 calories, 6 g fiber

Also, please note that although some of these differences don't seem very big compared to others, they add up to be quite significant over time—and especially when we make multiple small changes. I mean, just imagine the difference if we made the switch on every one of these foods!

> We would be much thinner if we all just made this one simple change.

One obvious baby step that's been discussed in this book has been eating frequently versus fewer, bigger meals. Sometimes this is much easier said than done. Here are some examples of important steps to make to ensure that you are eating frequently (that is, when you're hungry!).

The Breakfast Police

I honestly wish there were such an institution! Americans would be so much thinner if we all just made this one simple change! It's seems so easy to do— and has such wonderful consequences. One friend of mine lost seven pounds in a month just from making this one change: eating breakfast every morning whereas she didn't before.

However, I know that for those of us who have to rise early in the morning, this isn't always as easy as it seems. Either we don't have enough time, or it's so early we're not even hungry yet! I know from experience how that feels. But here's a trick that worked great for me: breakfast smoothies! Because I often had to be at work by 7 A.M., I had no time or appetite before leaving the house. What I did was make a fruit smoothie out of a variety (depending on the day) of fresh or frozen fruit, soy yogurt or soy ice cream, and juice or almond milk. I'd just throw it all in the blender the night before and keep it in the fridge over night in a big thermo-mug! The next day I would take my smoothie to work (or class) with me and slowly sip it over the course of the morning. It was funny how I was literally "eating" my breakfast while other people thought I was drinking coffee!

> I was "eating" my breakfast while other people thought I was drinking coffee.

Another simple way to slip breakfast in is to bring a couple pieces of fruit (or dried fruit) and a high fiber granola or health bar with you and snack as you work. If you can get away with chewing as you work, this is a great option!

If you already eat breakfast, but want to eat when you're hungry more, I suggest you get in the wonderful habit of bringing food with you—wherever you go. Stash some trail mix, dried fruit, nuts, or seeds (all of which have a naturally long shelf life and are very high-fiber) everywhere you find yourself frequently: your car, your locker at the gym or school, your desk, and definitely your house! Even your purse will do! Start scheduling in snack times when you've found yourself formerly suppressing your appetite (usually late morning and afternoons). Let your coffee break, or your time between classes or driving commute, become a snack break—but only when you're hungry!

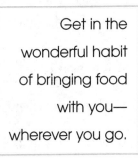

Get in the wonderful habit of bringing food with you— wherever you go.

What about eating out? Let's be honest, everyone eats out, and we shouldn't completely rule this pleasure out of our lives. I love to dine out when it's a nice restaurant. But many of us don't eat out because we love it, but because we have no other choice: there's no food at home and we didn't bring lunch with us. The good news is, this can be completely changed!

Making the Time

You know how everyone always says that if we really want to do something, we will make the time? Well, this is one area that is absolutely worth the extra time: it's your health and body we're talking about here. When we just plan a little more ahead: by writing down what we need from the store and actually shopping for it, by cooking our meals ourselves (remember: always cook at least four meals' worth so you have your own "fast food" at home), and by bringing that food with us for lunch the next day,

> This is one area that is absolutely worth the extra time.

we are making a wise investment. Not only will that save us a tremendous amount of money from not eating out as often, but we will eat healthier, lose weight, and feel way, way better.

One baby step you may want to make is to simply count how many times a week you currently eat out, and decrease that number

> Count how many times a week you currently eat out, and decrease that number by one or two.

by once or twice a week. Again, because restaurant and fast-food portion sizes are so big, because the food itself is generally very low in fiber (and other nutrients) and high in calories, any change you make is going to make a tremendous difference. Maybe you'll even come to the place where eating out is a treat—a special occasion that you really appreciate—instead of the place where "there's no other option"!

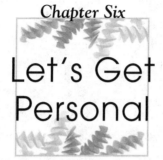

Chapter Six

Let's Get Personal

**_Personalizing Your Own Baby Steps
and Making Them Reality!_**

I sincerely hope that by now you are inspired to make a bunch of baby steps in your eating plan. But I want to take this time to remind you that in order for them to work, they must be *permanent*. Therefore, I recommend one baby step at a time. Set yourself up for success by starting with one that's easiest for you. The best way to do this is to pick one change you know you can make over the long run, and implement it until you reach the point that you've forgotten you ever made a change! In other words, don't make another baby step until the first one feels natural to you and you don't feel the least bit deprived.

For example, instead of swearing you'll never drink another soda again, when currently you drink three or more a day, pace yourself by committing to drink one less soda a day for three weeks. At the end of three weeks, toss out another soda a day, until ultimately, you only drink water… but it's now natural to you. Get the picture? I like the time frame of three weeks because it's long enough to enable us to make permanent changes, but short enough to keep moving with the baby steps. If it seems that this is too long or short of a time for some of the changes you want to make, try adding or subtracting a week's time—but again, remember that permanent weight loss takes time, so be patient with yourself.

> Permanent weight loss takes time, so be patient with yourself.

Why don't you write down six baby steps that you want to make, and order them from what you predict to be the easiest to least easy (of course, they should all be relatively easy for you):

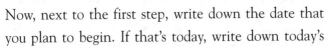

_____

_____

_____

_____

_____

_____

Now, next to the first step, write down the date that you plan to begin. If that's today, write down today's date! Then, from whatever date you've chosen for the first step, write down the date three weeks from that day for your second baby step, three weeks later for the third, and so on. Mark all these dates in your calendar.

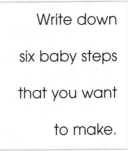

Write down

six baby steps

that you want

to make.

Once you reach the three-week date for each step, contemplate how comfortable you are at that point before you add another change to your diet plan. If you feel good, then go for it. If you find that you feel somewhat deprived, then take another week before making a new change. If at the end of a month it still feels unnatural, then choose a new step to make—one that is more natural to your lifestyle. Do this until you have successfully implemented all six baby steps. At that time, you might want to just enjoy your new eating patterns or you might want to make some more changes. Just remember, no matter how enthusiastic you are: this isn't a diet, it's a lifetime change, so don't go overboard! You have the rest of your life to do it!

Blessings to you!

The UnDiet
Order Form

Mail orders: 3104 "O" St. #259
Sacramento, CA 95816

Telephone orders: 916-736-2337

E-mail orders: schwags@cwia.com

Please send *The UnDiet* to:

Name: _____

Address: _____

City: _____ State: _____

Zip: _____

Telephone: (_____) _____

Book Price: $8.99

Shipping: $3.00 for the first book and $1.00 for each additional book to cover shipping and handling within US, Canada, and Mexico. International orders add $6.00 for the first book and $2.00 for each additional book.